DR. SEBI

MUCUS

CLEANSE

Easy Guide & Action Plan For Natural
Mucus Removal, Full-body Detox,
Liver Cleanse, High Blood Pressure, &
Diabetes Reversal Through Dr. Sebi
Alkaline Diet Approved Herbs And
Products

Shobi Nolan

Contents

to Prevent/CleanseExcess Mucus

CHAPTER 4

Dr Sebi Food List

OTHER BOOK BY THE SAME AUTHOR

CHAPTER 1

Introduction

Dr. Sebi's alkaline diet is a plant-based diet that helps to eliminate toxic wastes from the body and rejuvenate body cells.

The alkaline diet relies strictly on a list of plant foods and products approved by Dr. Sebi. Through his diet, Dr. Sebi did great wonders in people's lives; cured many diseases and revived complicated health conditions. In fact, it is one of the best plant-based diets. It was listed as one of the most popular diets in 2019.

If we can eat delicious meals and free our body from diseases, what again are we looking for? Dr. Sebi's diet can help you detox your body completely, including mucus removal, liver cleansing, diabetes reversal, cancer treatment, lupus and herpes cure, etc. Learn how to eat good foods, and you may not need medications to stay healthy.

In this book, you will learn all the simple steps you need to detox your body completely and keep it free from excess mucus. You don't need medications to cleanse mucus from your body when you can easily get rid of it naturally by drinking and eating the right foods. These foods can be found in the nearest local grocery store.

Prepare your mind and stock your kitchen with the list of foods you will get in this book. Then follow the action plans and steps designed for any of the intracellular cleansing methods with Dr. Sebi's approved herbs.

But before we get started, let's look at;

- Dr. Sebi and his diet.
- Mucus and your health.

Who is Dr. Sebi?

Alfredo Darlington Bowman is an African herbalist who developed an alkaline plant diet that is based on bio-mineral balance theory. Though he is not a certified medical doctor or a Ph.D. holder, he is widely known as Dr. Sebi.

His diet is named after his popular name, The Dr. Sebi Diet. His diet was developed for those that wish to naturally detox their body for total wellness and prevent diseases by eating approved healthy plant foods.

Dr. Sebi claimed that our body is protected from diseases when it is in an alkaline state. According to him, acidic state of the body and mucus buildup in the body are the major causes of various diseases.

Though there is no scientific backup, Dr. Sebi claimed that his diet has the potential to cure lupus, sickle cell anemia, AIDS, and leukemia. He believes his diet could completely restore alkalinity in the body and detoxify the whole body.

Dr. Sebi Alkaline Diet

Dr. Sebi's diet is regarded as a vegan diet since it is a completely plant-based diet. No animal product is allowed in the diet.

Dr. Sebi claimed that this diet can make the body heal itself completely from diseases. Though there is no scientific proof for this, a lot of people who are on the diet have attested to the claim.

As a result, Dr. Sebi's diet is ranked one of the most popular diets in 2019.

The Dr. Sebi Diet Guide

Dr. Sebi's diet is solely based on plants and supplements approved by Dr. Sebi.

The diet guide can be found on his website. The simple rules to follow on Dr. Sebi diet are;

- Only foods and products listed in the nutritional guide are to be consumed.
- You must drink at least 1 gallon of water every day (that is about 3.8 liters).
- If you are on any medication, you have to take your Dr. Sebi supplements, at least, one hour before your medication.
- You don't take alcohol.

- You must not eat any animal products.

- Don't use the microwave to prepare your foods.

- Only consume naturally grown grains as listed in the guide. No wheat product is allowed.

- No seedless fruit and no canned food are permitted.

Moreover, you are expected to be using Dr. Sebi's supplements to support your diet.

Why You Need Dr. Sebi Diet

Dr. Sebi's diet has so many benefits as claimed by Dr. Sebi. Just like other plant-based diets, no scientific research has backed up any health benefit claims. But many users of the diet guide have also claimed that the diet is good and works perfectly as claimed.

Some of the potential health benefits of Dr. Sebi diet include but not limited to;

- Weight loss
- Prevention of heart disease
- Liver cleansing
- Mucus cleansing
- Cancer prevention
- Eye protection

- Immune boost
- Skin protection and maintenance
- Diabetes treatment and prevention
- Healthy bone formation, etc.

Possible Health Implications of Dr. Sebi Diet

Though Dr. Sebi's diet has a lot of health benefits attached to it, there are some things to consider before starting the diet.

Highly Restrictive:

Dr. Sebi's diet is one of the most difficult diets to live on. It is only based on selected plant-based foods and supplements. Though it's plant-based, not all plant foods are approved. So, to be on this diet, one has to go through the food guidelines and stick with the approved herbs, fruits, and veggies.

Vitamin B-12 Deficiency:

Animal products are the only sources of vitamin B-12. This literally means that Dr. Sebi diet contains no vitamin B-12 which is highly vital for blood cells, nerves, and development of DNA. Though the high availability of folic acid in the diet can help to cover up some side effects of vitamin B-12 deficiency, it can as well worsen the situation.

To avoid the risk of vitamin B-12 deficiency, which is common among older people and kids, it is advisable to take vitamin B-12 supplements along with the diet. This helps the body to produce healthy red blood cells and prevents the risk of anemia.

Protein

Plant foods like lentils, beans, and soy

with high amounts of protein contents are not approved in the Dr. Sebi diet. Due to the high restriction of plant foods in the Dr. Sebi diet, it is always difficult to get enough protein from the diet.

Protein is a very important compound in the body that helps to keep the brain, hormones, DNA, bones, and muscles healthy and functional. Lack of protein in the body can lead to many health complications. To stay on Dr. Sebi's diet, one needs to eat a lot of plant foods to be able to get much-needed protein for the body.

Omega-3 Fatty Acids

Research suggests that plant foods are not the major sources of omega-3 fatty acids. This may be an issue for anyone on a restricted plant-based diet. But anyone on the Dr. Sebi diet may consider taking a lot of walnuts and hemp seeds as they are good sources of omega-3 fatty acids.

Note: It is highly advisable that you consult your doctor first before starting any new diet.

NOTE

CHAPTER 2

Mucus Cleanse

Everything You Need to Know

Mucus is an aqueous secretion produced by the cells of the mucous glands. It serves as a covering for the mucous membranes. Mucus is mainly composed of water, which is the mucin secretions.

It is an important element of the epithelial lining fluid, the airway surface liquid, which is the lining of the respiratory tract. Mucus helps to protect the lungs during breathing by trapping foreign particles and infectious agents like dust, allergens, virus, bacteria, etc.

The human body always tends to

produce more mucus in order to protect and prevent the airway tissues from drying out. Thus, there is a continuous production of mucus in the respiratory system.

When foreign objects get trapped by the mucus, the mucus becomes thick and changes color most of the time. This thick mucus that is usually coughed out as sputum is known as phlegm.

Mucus also plays an important role in the digestive system. The layer formed by the mucus in the small intestine and colon helps to protect the intestinal epithelial cells from bacterial infections. It also serves as a lubricant for movement of foods through the esophagus.

Interestingly, mucus is the body's

natural lubricant in females which helps during sexual intercourse. It also helps to fight against infection in the reproductive system.

Mucus And Body Health

There is a continuous process of mucus production in the body, which helps to protect the body systems from infections and also provides necessary lubrication to the body.

Thus, the presence of mucus in our body is important. When mucus traps foreign and infectious bodies, it becomes phlegm. Phlegm and excess mucus in the body is not healthy. As the body produces up to a liter of mucus every day, it is vital to get rid of it to keep the body healthy.

Accumulation of mucus in the

body is the major cause of illnesses as claimed by Dr. Sebi. So, excess mucus can be a red flag for unhealthy state of the body.

Causes Of Mucus Buildup in The Body:

Just like in snails and other animals that secrete mucus, there are triggers for the production of mucus. In human beings, the major triggers are dryness and inflammation of the body. Some factors that may lead to dryness, inflammation, and other mucus secretion triggers are;

- Dry air (environment)
- Smoking
- Allergies
- Infections
- Acid reflux

- Asthma
- Low water/liquid consumption
- Medications etc.

These factors and more contribute to excess buildup of mucus in the body. The body naturally produces mucus to ensure that foreign objects (toxic and/or infectious) don't interact with the body cells. The more we have these foreign bodies, the more the body produces mucus. When these objects get trapped by the mucus, the mucus becomes thick and builds up as phlegm.

Moreover, our body must stay lubricated for swift movement of particles and cells in the body. Thus, dryness of the body makes the body produce more mucus, which is the liquid the body can produce naturally.

Mucus Natural Cleanse - The Dr. Sebi Way

If you are on the Dr Sebi Diet, below are simple steps you can take to clear out and prevent excess mucus and still maintain the diet recommendations.

Hydration:

Enough liquid in the body, especially warm liquid can help drain the sinuses and thin the mucus. Thus, drinking high amounts of water can help clear out mucus from the body.

Dr Sebi recommends high intake of water. Also, most fruits and vegetables recommended by Dr Sebi diet have high water content. These foods help to keep the body hydrated and prevent excess mucus production.

Moreover, some drinks like coffee and alcohol can cause dehydration in the body. Anyone on the Dr Sebi diet must stay away from alcohol. This helps to avoid dehydration.

Action:

Take a lot of water, smoothies, and juice made with Dr Sebi approved foods.

Expectorant:

Expectorant is known to help in clearing mucus. Expectorant loosens and thins mucus, which makes it easy to cough it out of the system.

There are some herbs in the Dr Sebi diet which can serve as expectorants. The major and most used herb in the Dr Sebi approved herbs is the Red Clover.

Red Clover is a super healthy herb which aids circulation in the body. It is a natural blood purifier, and also serves as an expectorant. It is widely used by women in treating menopause related conditions like hot flashes and lumbar spine protection.

So, taking red clover can help to loosen and clear mucus from the body.

Action:

In 8 oz of hot water, steep 1 - 2 teaspoons of the dried flower and allow for up to 30 minutes. Then drink at least 2 and not more than 3 cups per day.

Or sip 1ml of the fluid extract with hot

water three times daily.

Essential Oils:

Some essential oils have been proposed to be very effective in the treatment of lung disease related symptoms. People use essential oils for the treatment and prevention of chest cold and sinusitis. Some of these essential oils can be gotten from Dr Sebi approved products like eucalyptus, oregano, and thyme.

Eucalyptus has been widely used for many years to treat coughs and reduce mucus production. It helps to loosen the mucus so it can be easily coughed out. Thus, it relieves nagging coughs.

Action:

Make your own homemade vapor rub by adding 12 drops of eucalyptus oil to ¼ cup of coconut oil. Alternatively, add 1 drop of eucalyptus oil to 1 teaspoon of water.

First test the mixture to know whether it is safe for use. Then apply it directly on your skin, especially on your throat and chest. This makes the scents to easily reach the nose and mouth.

Note: These recommendations are for adults alone.

7-Day Plan to Cleanse Mucus Completely

The methods we have discussed truly help to cleanse the mucus from the body. But the result might not be a fast as we want it.

However, we can catalyze the process and make it faster. Yes, we can cleanse mucus as soon as we desire, depending on the program we follow. But before you follow any program, consult your health professional. Remember, the developer of any health program only gives you what works for him or her.

They do not know your health condition. So, they use the health condition they know as a standard or reference.

Do your due diligence and consult your doctor first.

This 7-day mucus cleanse program is highly effective. All you need is three types of drinks. You can take otherjuice and smoothies, but do not skip these ones during the program. In addition to that, you will also do breathing exercise first thing in the morning and last thing before you sleep in the night.

Here are the program details.

- Every morning, do 5-10 minutes of breathing exercise upon arising.
- Then drink 16 ounce of prune juice.
- Drink grape juice throughout the day, especially after lunch.

- Eat your dinner before 7pm every day. About 15 minutes later, drink 3-4 tablespoons of onion water. Grate the onion and soak in water around noon, so it can stay in the water for about 7-8 hours before use.

- Finally, do another 5 minutes of breathing exercise before you sleep.

- Righteously follow this simple program for 7 days. Then let us know your experience after the 7th day.

Other Possible Cleansing Methods

- Research suggests that taking a lot of high fiber content foods may help to treat respiratory issues that are linked to phlegm. There are loads of fiber rich foods in Dr Sebi diet.

- Capsaicin in cayenne may help to thin and clear out sinuses temporarily. This gets the mucus to move easily.

- Research suggests that drinks and foods that contain ginger can help to clear excess mucus and treat cough.

- Gargling with warm salt water may not only kill germs. It can help to remove mucus that accumulates on the back of our throat.

Note:

Mucus is not a bad substance in our body. It is a very vital element in the system as we have discussed its roles in the body. So, having it does not mean illness.

Where we are much concerned is having excess or accumulation of this liquid in our body systems. Accumulation of it is not good for the body and may lead to various diseases.

But before you take any action regarding mucus, or any health-related issue in your body, consult your doctor first.

If you are a woman and you want to burst that mucus in three days, then you don't want to miss **Dr.**

Sebi Approved 3-Day Mucus Buster Diet for Women

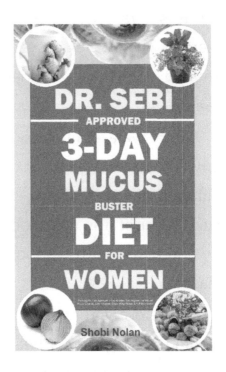

Link to kindle edition:

https://www.amazon.com/dp/B08GMBD8DX

Link to print edition:

pg. 30

https://www.amazon.com/APPROVED-3-DAY-MUCUS-BUSTER-WOMEN/dp/B08GVJTRNY

NOTE

CHAPTER 3

Dr Sebi Approved Vegetables to Prevent/Cleanse Excess Mucus

Foods with high water content and/or fiber can help the body stay hydrated, and hence prevent and cleanse excess mucus in the body. The Dr. Sebi vegetables are awesome foods with high amount of water and fiber content.

Taking these veggies will not only help you cleanse mucus; they will help your body to detox and heal naturally.

Below are some of the veggies and ways you can add them to your diet for a super healthy living.

Tomato (The Plum and Cherry)

Scientific Name: *Solanum lycopersicum*

Overview

Tomato is a popular plant grown all over the world in a temperate climate. It's widely used in different cuisines. Though it's native to western South America, China, India, the United States, and Turkey are currently the highest producers of tomatoes.

Tomato is used in many ways because of its umami flavor. It can be taken raw or cooked.

Major Compounds

Beta-carotene, lutein zeaxanthin, thiamine, niacin, vitamin B-6, vitamin

C, vitamin E, vitamin K, magnesium, manganese, phosphorus, potassium

Health benefits

Heart health: Tomatoes contain high amounts of potassium and fiber. These components are important for keeping the heart healthy. Fiber helps the body to reduce cholesterol level in the blood. High consumption of potassium helps to lower the blood pressure which is good for the heart.

Healthy bone: Phosphorus, magnesium, and vitamin C play crucial roles in the development of string and healthy bones. Tomatoes contain high amounts of phosphorus and moderate amounts of magnesium and vitamin C.

Eye health: The lutein and beta-carotene found in tomatoes are needed by our eyes to protect the retina and keep the eye free from macular degeneration.

Prevents cancer: tomatoes contain several vitamins and antioxidants such as lycopene, beta-carotene, vitamin C, etc. These components have properties that enables them to fight cancer cells and free radicals that can cause damage to the body cells.

How To Use

Tomatoes are used in many ways. It can be eaten raw or cooks. It can be used to make side dishes. Awesome for fruit and vegetable salads. Tomorrow is the major ingredient for stew. Many use it to cook soup, make sandwiches, or add it to wraps.

There are so many ways to use it. It can be used for smoothies and juice.

Nutrition fact

Per 100g

- Calories: 18 kcal
- Carbs: 3.9g
- Sugars: 2.6g
- Fiber: 1.2g
- Fat: 0.2g
- Protein: 0.9g

Side Effects

Excessive intake of tomatoes can lead to some unhealthy conditions. Some of these side effects include diarrhea, acid reflux, headache, kidney stones, lycopenodermia, joint pain, severe throat/mouth irritation, vomiting, mild spasms, dizziness, etc.

NOTE

Squash

Scientific Name: *Cucurbita spp.*

Overview

Squash is a widely used food crop that originated from Mexico. Now popular in the South, North America, and Asia. India and China have been the highest producers of squash so far.

There are different types of squashes with several color variations. Squash has fed many mouths and is still feeding a lot at the moment. It is cooked and used in different dishes.

Major Compounds

Beta-carotene, lutein, zeaxanthin, thiamine, riboflavin, niacin, pantothenic acid, vitamin B6, folate, vitamin C, vitamin K, iron, magnesium, manganese, phosphorus, potassium, zinc, oleic, palmitic, and linoleic fatty acids.

Health benefits

Heart health: Fiber and potassium are important substances that help to take care of the heart. High fiber content foods help to reduce the cholesterol level in our blood. Enough intake of potassium helps the body to lower blood pressure.

Squash contains a high amount of potassium which is vital to the heart.

Cancer: squash contains important antioxidants that may help the body to prevent cancer. Some of these antioxidants reduce the growth rate of cancer cells and help to protect the body cells against free radicals.

Healthy Eye: Squash contains beta-carotene and lutein, which are important compounds for healthy eyes. They help to protect the retina and keep the eyes free from macular degeneration.

How To Use

Simply wash and peel off the skin. Then use as you desire. You can cook your squash, or roast it. Smashed and used as an ingredient for other dishes like soup.

Some squash has tough cover. To peel them off you need to put them in your oven for about 2 minutes, with the skin pierced with a fork. Or bake/cook with the skin on. Then it will be easier to remove the skin.

Nutrition fact

Per 100g

- Calories: 16 kcal
- Carbs: 3.4g
- Sugars: 2.2g
- Fiber: 1.1g
- Fat: 0.2g
- Protein: 1.2g

Side Effects

Some of the side effects associated with the use of squash include allergic reactions such as dermatitis, itching, difficulty in breathing, nasal congestion, swelling of face and lips, etc.

NOTE

Onion

Scientific Name: *Allium cepa*

Overview

Onion is one of the most popular food ingredients used worldwide. Though its origin has many claims, the only fact is that onion originated from Asia.

It is widely cultivated all over the world. It can be eaten raw or cooked. Onion can be pungent to the eye when exposed. Three types of onions are predominant; the yellow onion, red onion, and white onion. All are flavorful and super healthy for use.

Major Compounds

Polyphenols, thiamine, riboflavin, niacin, pantothenic acid, vitamin B-6, folate, vitamin C, calcium, iron, magnesium, manganese, phosphorus, potassium, zinc

Health benefits

Cancer: the antioxidants in onions can help the body to fight against cancer by protecting the body cells against oxidative damage. They can reduce the growth of cancer cells, and thus, helps to reduce the risk of cancer.

Heart health: fiber in our foods helps to lower the level of cholesterol in our body. Moreover, the high amount of potassium in onions plays a vital role in the reduction of blood pressure. These properties of onions plus more ensure a healthy heart.

Osteoporosis: Calcium, potassium, and vitamin C are important to the bone. These compounds provided in good amounts by onion can help the body to develop strong and healthy bones.

Anti-inflammatory: Destroying radical cells that are toxic to the body is one of the means our body uses to prevent inflammation. The antioxidants from onions help the body to fight against these radicals.

How To Use

Onion is used to prepare most dishes. First peel off the outer layer and wash. Dice or slice to your taste and add to your food; salads, wraps, sandwiches, soup, stew, etc. It can be taken raw or cooked. Anyway, it is super healthy for consumption.

Nutrition fact

Per 100g

- Calories: 40
- Fat: 0.1g
- Carbs: 9g
- Fiber: 1.7g
- Sugar: 4.2g
- Protein: 1.1g

Side Effects

Some of the side effects associated with the use of onions include blurred vision, dermatitis, bronchial asthma, itching, sweating, and anaphylaxis

NOTE

Olive

Scientific Name: *Olea europaea*

Overview

Dominant in the Mediterranean region, olive is a very important ingredient in the Mediterranean foods. It has wonderful health benefits. Some people claim that it is the healthiest food on earth and one of the oldest known trees, thanks to its religious attachment.

Though olive is not native to the Americas, it is one of the most popular ingredients used in America, especially the oil.

Major Compounds

potassium, calcium, magnesium,

vitamin E, phosphorus, sodium,
polyphenol, iron, choline

Health benefits

Heart health: olive contains
carbohydrates that are mostly made
up of fiber. This high fiber content of
olive helps the body to lower
cholesterol levels.

Diabetes: research suggests that food
with high fiber content strongly helps
to reduce blood sugar levels. Olive is a
good source of fiber and consuming a
good amount of olive will help prevent
and possibly treat type 2 diabetes.

Anti-inflammatory: olive contains
wonderful compounds and antioxidants

that help to protect the body cells against oxidative damages, which may lead to inflammation of the body.

Cancer: the antioxidants provided by olive helps to reduce the growth of cancer cells in the body. Thus, taking olive can help one to prevent cancer cell formation.

How To Use

Olive is cultivated for different use. But most people cultivate olive for its oil which is the most used oil in the Mediterranean diet.

Nutrition fact

Per 100 g

- Calories: 146 kcal

- Carbs: 3.84g

- Sugars: 0.54g

- Fiber: 3.3g

- Fat: 15.32g

- Protein: 1.03g

Side Effects

There is no enough record on the side
effects of olive. But there could be
possible allergic reactions. If you have
a complicated health condition, consult
your physician before use.

NOTE

Okra

Scientific Name: *Abelmoschus esculentus*

Overview

Okra is a widely used vegetable all over the world. Some regions call it Okro or ladies' finger. This healthy plant that originated from West Africa has a mucilaginous property. This makes most foods cooked with okra to be slimy, unless it's deslimed. One of the things mostly used to deslime okra is tomato.

This healthy vegetable is widely cultivated for food because of its nutritional values. It is used in many ways such as in making salads, soups, stews, etc.

Major Compounds

Protein, carbohydrates, fiber, vitamin K, vitamin C, thiamin, folate, magnesium, riboflavin, niacin, potassium, calcium, iron, phosphorus, zinc, flavonoids, and isoquercetin

Health benefits

Prevention of Cancer: okra contains lectin and folate. Researchers suggest that these compounds strongly inhibit the gowth of cancer cells. Thus, taking enough okra can help one to prevent the risk of cancer.

Pregnancy: The folate gotten from okra helps to keep a healthy pregnancy. Lack of folate in the body may possibly lead to miscarriage.

Prevents diabetes: Test done on animals (rat) shows that okra can reduce the fat and blood sugar level in the body.

Heart health: Okra provides the body with useful fibers which can help to keep the heart-healthy. American Heart Association (AHA) suggests that food with high fiber content helps the body to reduce cholesterol level.

Osteoporosis: okra provides a high amount of calcium and vitamin K to the body. Calcium and vitamin K are very vital for the development of strong and healthy bones.

How To Use

Okra can be used in many ways. It can be taken raw, roasted, pickled, fried, boiled, or sauteed. You can add it to your soup, salads, or other foods.

To remove the sliminess of okra in your food, try and cook it over high heat and avoid cooking in a crowded pot.

You can also pickle it or cook with acidic food like tomato.

Nutrition fact

Per 100g

- Calories: 33
- Fat: 0.2g
- Carbs: 7g
- Fiber: 3.2g
- Sugar: 1.5g

- Protein: 1.9g

Side Effects

Some side effects associated with the use of okra include cramping, diarrhea, gas, and bloating.

NOTE

Nopals

Scientific Name: *Opuntia spp.*

Overview

Native to Mexico, nopales is a food ingredient with important health benefits. There are about 114 species of nopales in Mexico. This highly medicinal food is not popular like other herbs such as lettuces, kale, etc, but it is common among the residents of southwest America.

It's popularly known in English as "prickly pear".

Major Compounds

Manganese, vitamin C, magnesium, calcium, antioxidants, sodium, potassium

Health benefits

Antiviral: research suggests that nopales gas antiviral properties that can be used against herpes and HIV.

Antioxidant: Nopales have a high content of antioxidants which help to protect the body cells against radical damage and reduce oxidative stress.

Blood Sugar Level: research has it that nopales have important properties that can help to regulate blood sugar levels.

Cholesterol: earlier studies suggest that nopales can lower cholesterol levels, especially LDL cholesterol.

Enlarged Prostate: Nopales may help to reduce enlarged prostate, which is a serious health condition for men. It may as well help to treat prostate cancer.

How To Use

Nopales can be eaten raw or cooked. It can be used to make juice, jams, smoothies, tea, etc.

It can be prepared with other Dr. Sebi approved foods as side dishes, salads, etc.

Nutrition fact

Per 100g

- Calories: 16
- Total Fat: 0.1g

- Fiber: 2g

- Sugar: 1.1g

- Protein: 1.4g

Side Effects

Some of the side effects associated with nopales include bloating, headache, diarrhea, nausea

NOTE

Mushrooms

Scientific Name: *Agaricus bisporus*

Overview

With over 14,000 types, mushrooms are widely cultivated all over the world for commercial and medicinal use. China, Italy, and the United States are known to be among the highest producers of mushrooms.

The most consumed mushroom until this century remains the white mushrooms. There are many health benefits associated with mushrooms and that is one of the major reasons why it gained its popularity.

However, not all mushrooms are edible as some can be highly toxic to the body. There are over 2,000 edible mushrooms. Among the edible ones, shiitake is not approved for the Dr Sebi diet. So, it's pertinent that one should avoid shitake and any other mushroom that is not edible.

Major Compounds

Protein, pantothenic acid, riboflavin, niacin, copper, calcium, selenium, potassium, fiber, vitamin D, ergothioneine, glutathione

Health benefits

Cancer Prevention: The antioxidants in mushrooms can help to prevent cancer cells from reproducing. Thus, mushrooms help the body to lower the risk of cancer.

**Neurodegenerative Disease
(Alzheimer's)**: Ergothioneine and
glutathione which are majorly
produced by mushrooms are claimed to
be potentially useful for the treatment
of Alzheimer's and Parkinson's
diseases

Heart Health: Mushrooms are one of
the major producers of potassium.
High intake of potassium helps to
reduce blood pressure.

Diabetes: The fiber content of
mushrooms can help to fight against
diabetes. Fiber is known to be useful in
managing type 2 diabetes.

How To Use

First trim the end of the stalk, clean, and wash before use. It can be sliced, diced, or used the whole. Though it can be taken raw, cooked mushrooms are most preferred.

Mushrooms can be used to make salads, side dishes, pizza, scrambles, quiche, omelet, sandwiches, wraps, etc.

Nutrition fact

Per 100g

- Calories: 22
- Fat: 0.3g
- Total Carbs: 3.3g
- Fiber: 1g
- Sugar: 2g
- Protein: 3.1g

Side Effects

Dryness of the mouth or throat, rashes, diarrhea, itchiness, stomach upset, cramps, headache, nausea, vomiting, and diarrhea

NOTE

Dandelion

Scientific Name: *Taraxacum officinale*

Overview

Dandelion is an herbaceous plant grown all over the world for food and medicinal purposes. It's claimed to have a myriad of medicinal properties that can be used in the prevention and potential cure for physical ailments.

Native to North America and Eurasia, dandelion is widely consumed as a nutritious food. All parts of the plant are edible, including the flower, leaves, roots, and stems.

The flowers are known to contain high amounts of phytochemicals, with the leaves rich in lutein, while the root has a lot of probiotic fibers.

Major Compounds

Vitamin A, folate, vitamin K, vitamin C, calcium, potassium, iron, manganese, polyphenols, inulin, lutein, beta-carotene

Health benefits

Good Source of Antioxidants:
dandelion provides the body with a good number of antioxidants such as beta-caroteneand polyphenols which help to protect the body cells against radical damages.

Regulation of Cholesterol Levels:
researches done on animals suggests that dandelion is very effective in reducing cholesterol levels. It also

lowers the amount of fat in the liver, which means that dandelion can be used for the treatment of fatty liver disease.

Blood Sugar Regulation: the antihyperglycemic, anti-inflammatory and antioxidative properties found in dandelion can be useful for the treatment of type 2 diabetes.

Anti-inflammatory: chemical extracts from dandelion are claimed to be potent in the reduction of body inflammation.

Blood Pressure Regulation: potassium is known to be an effective supplement for lowering blood pressure.

pg. 76

Weight Loss: the chlorogenic acid found in dandelion can be effective in reducing weight and lipid accumulation.

Prevention of Cancer: Research suggests that dandelion can be highly effective in the prevention of cancer as it has the potential to inhibit the growth of cancer cells.

Immune System Boost: The antibacterial and antiviral properties of dandelion can be useful for the immune system. Research suggests that dandelion can inhibit the growth of hepatitis B.

How To Use

Dandelion can be used in many ways. Depending on how you want it, it's mostly preferred when blanched to remove some bitterness. It can be taken raw (both fresh and dried), added to smoothies, teas, and juice, or used to make salads. It can be added to soup. The root can be roasted and used as coffee.

Nutrition fact

Per 100g

- Calories: 45
- Total Fat: 0.7g
- Total Carbs: 9.2g
- Fiber: 3.5g
- Sugar: 0.7g
- Protein: 2.7g

Side Effects

There is no enough record on the side effect on the use of dandelions. But dandelion can cause allergic reactions, diarrhea, or heartburn.

NOTE

Lettuce

Scientific Name: *Lactuca sativa*

Overview

Lettuce which originated from Egypt and mostly produced in China is widely known for its wonderful health benefits. Some people call it the perfect weight-loss food.

It can be used in diverse ways for various purposes, especially for medicinal purposes. In many regions, it is used for the treatment of typhoid, body pain, smallpox, rheumatism, coughs, and nervousness - even insanity, though there is no scientific backup for this claim.

There are different types of lettuce which include leaf lettuce, romaine lettuce, iceberg, summercrip, butterhead, red leaf, oilseed, and celtuce.

Note: Iceberg is not approved by Dr. Sebi.

Major Compounds

Vitamin K, vitamin A (beta-carotene, lutein, zeaxanthin), folate, iron, thiamine, riboflavin, pantothenic acid, vitamin c, vitamin e, calcium, magnesium, manganese, phosphorus, potassium, sodium, zinc

Health benefits

Prevents Dehydration: lettuce, especially red lettuce is made up of 96% water. This can help to keep the body hydrated.

Antioxidant: lettuce contains a lot of antioxidants such as beta-carotene which helps to protect the body cells against radical damage. Antioxidants play vital roles in the wholesome wellness of our bodies.

Heart Health: the presence of potassium in lettuce may help to lower the level of blood pressure.

Eye Health: The beta-carotene and other antioxidants got from lettuce help to protect the eye from macular degeneration.

Prevents Diabetes: Lettuce has a

low glycemic index and zero glycemic loads which are good for those trying to lower their blood sugar, especially for managing type 2 diabetes.

How To Use

First wash the lettuce, pound on a chopping board to make it soft. Separate the leaves and dry. Then tear into smaller parts and dress.

Lettuce can be used to make smoothies, salads, and sandwiches. It can also be added to soups and wraps.

Nutrition fact

Per 100g

- Calories: 15
- Fat: 0.2g
- Carbs: 2.9g

- Fiber: 1.3g

- Sugar: 0.8g

- Protein: 1.4g

Side Effects

Some of the potential side effects associated with lettuce consumption include sweating, itching, fast heartbeat, nausea, vomiting, pupil dilation, diarrhea, dizziness, ringing in the ears, vision rashes, vision changes, sedation, and breathing difficulty.

NOTE

Izote

Scientific Name: *Yucca gigantea*

Overview

Commonly known as yucca, izote is a garden plant that is native to Central America and Mexico. It is claimed to have varieties of medicinal properties. It is one of the most popular sources of saponin, a natural detergent.

Generally, it is cultivated as a houseplant, ornamental garden, herb, or food. Thus, it is used in diverse ways, especially in the treatment of illness like arthritis.

Though it can survive in different soils and conditions, it thrives most in hot semi-arid or warm climates.

Health benefits

Arthritis: According to research, the chemical extracts from izotes can potentially help in the treatment of arthritis.

Heart Health: steroidal saponins from izote helps the body to lower cholesterol level in the blood. This helps to keep the heart healthy.

Prevention of Cancer: the phenols gotten from izote can help to prevent the growth of cancer cells, and thus, eliminating any potential risk of cancer.

Anti-inflammatory: izote contains

pg. 88

phenols like resveratrol and yuccaols A, B, C, D and E, which are known to be anti-inflammatory.

How To Use

First remove the ovaries and anthers. Then blanch for about 5 minutes. You can cook your izote with onion, tomatoes, and chili. Bool and eat with lemon juice, or use it with egg-battered patties.

Side Effects

Some possible side effects associated with izote are upset stomach, bitter taste, vomiting, nausea.

NOTE

Kale

Scientific Name: *Brassica oleracea*

Overview

Kale is one of the most popular veggies in the world. It is highly nutritious and heavily used for its medicinal properties.

It's claimed to originate from Asia Minor and Eastern Mediterranean where it was cultivated for food. Kale is best cultivated in the winter times for maximum yield.

Major Compounds

Protein, fiber, vitamins A, C, and K, folate, alpha-linolenic acid, lutein and zeaxanthin, phosphorus, potassium, calcium, zinc, carotenoids, phenols

Health benefits

Diabetes: The fiber content of kale can play an important role in the prevention and treatment of diabetes since fiber helps to regulate blood sugar level.

Antioxidants: kale contains a high amount of antioxidants which help to protect the body cells against oxidative damage.

Heart health: high intake of potassium and reduction in the consumption of sodium helps to lower the risk of high blood pressure. Moreover, fiber in our diet helps to lower cholesterol level. These properties help to take care of the heart.

Prevention Cancer: The presence of antioxidants in our body helps to protect our cells and hinder the development of cancer cells.

Healthy Eye: the lutein and zeaxanthin gotten from kale help to protect our eyes against macular degeneration. Vitamins, zinc, and beta-carotene help to protect the retina and keep the eyes healthy.

Healthy Bone: Calcium and vitamin K are very important for the development of healthy bones. Even, phosphorus and vitamin D also support the health of our bones.

Healthy skin and Hair: the human skin needs beta-carotene and vitamin A for development and maintenance of body tissues. Also, the vitamin C provided by kale helps to build and support the protein, collagen, responsible for skin and hair growth

How To Use

You can use kale in many ways. Kale can be eaten raw, steamed, or sauteed. Gently scrunch the kale leaf to make it soft. Then add it to your salads, sandwiches, and smoothies, wraps. Blend with other veggies and fruits to make

smoothies and juice. Saute with onion for a side dish. You can spice it up and bake for 15-30 minutes to make your kale chips.

pg. 94

Nutrition fact

Per 100g

- Calories: 49
- Fat: 0.9g
- Total Carbs: 9g
- Protein: 4.3g

Side Effects

If you are battling with hypothyroidism, kale is not the best vegetable for you. Consult your physician for your diets. Excessive intake of kale can inhibit the production of thyroid hormone.

NOTE

Garbanzo Beans

Scientific Name: *Cicer arietinum*

Overview

Garbanzo beans is a nutrient-dense legume which is highly cultivated almost in all parts of the world. It is highly rich in fiber, protein, folate, iron, etc.

There are two types of garbanzos, the big size with light color, which is predominant in the Americas and the small size with dark color that is mainly found in the Middle East and India

However, American garbanzo beans are far sweeter than the Indian garbanzo beans. This is one of those foods that takes time to cook, but it always comes out with great taste.

Major Compounds

Protein, folate, fiber, iron, phosphorus, fatty acids, sitosterol,

Health benefits

Diabetes: Beans are known to be slow in digestion. Garbanzo beans have a very low glycerin index (GI) and glycemic load (GL). These properties help to reduce blood sugar and insulin levels. Thus, it can be used to control the sugar level of patients with type 2 diabetes.

Heart Disease: the plant sterol in garbanzo beans known as sitosterol helps to lower the cholesterol level in the blood.

Obesity: the high fiber content of garbanzo beans can help to promote weight loss. High fiber content in a diet makes one have the feeling of fullness, and this satiating effect helps in weight loss.

How To Use

First sort the beans to remove stones and debris. Then soak overnight and cook for about 1 or 2 hours, depending on the heat you are using. Check for recipes and get directions. You can use the cooked garbanzo beans in many ways.

It can be added to your stew, soup, or salad. You can make hummus with it by blending it with olive oil, lemon juice, garlic, and tahini. Mashed and used in place of flour.

Roast and grind to make coffee.

Nutrition fact

Per 100g

- Calories: 378 kcal
- Carbs: 62.95g
- Sugars: 10.7g
- Fiber: 12.2g
- Fats: 6.04g
- Protein: 20.47g

Side Effects

Some of the side effects recorded on the use of garbanzo beans include stomach cramp, gas pains, and discomfort. The allergies associated include redness, rashes, inflammation, diarrhea, and hives.

NOTE

Cucumber

Scientific Name: *Cucumis sativus*

Overview

Cucumber is a creeping vine plant that is cultivated all over the world. According to history, cucumbers originated from India before spreading to other parts of the world.

It contains about 95% water which makes it one of the best fruits/vegetables to manage dehydration. It is cultivated for both food and medicinal purposes as it contains healthy substances that are highly beneficial to the body.

Major Compounds

Calcium, potassium, magnesium,

phosphorus, iron, sodium, vitamin C, beta-carotene, folate, lutein zeaxanthin, nantothenic acid, cucurbitacin, vitamin K, vitamin B-6, thiamine, riboflavin, niacin

Health benefits

Hydration: hydration is one of the major benefits of cucumber as it is made up of 95% water. This water is super healthy as it has important electrolytes which helps to prevent constipation and maintain healthy intestine.

Healthy Bone: vitamin and calcium are very important for the bone. Calcium keeps the bone strong and healthy while vitamin K facilitate the absorption of calcium. Also, vitamin D

pg. 104

supports the heath if the bone.

Cancer Prevention: Cucurbitacin is a nutrient know to inhibit cancer cells from reproducing and hence prevents the development of cancer cells.

Heart Health: The fiber content of cucumber helps to regulate cholesterol levels and prevent possible heart disease.

Diabetes Prevention: Cucumber has low glycerin index, which means it has low potential of increasing blood sugar. Also, according to American Heart Association (AHA), fiber helps to prevent type 2 diabetes.

How To Use

Cucumber is usually eaten raw. You can add it to your salads or sandwiches. Use it to make side dishes and have a good meal time. For your smoothies and juice, you can blend cucumber and add it.

There is no specific limitation to the use of cucumber. You can add it to any food you feel like enjoying with cucumber. The most important thing is for it to add value to your health and also give you a great taste.

Nutrition Facts

Per 100g

- Calories: 65 kJ (16 kcal)
- Carbs: 3.63g
- Sugars: 1.67

- Dietary fiber: 0.5 g
- Fat: 0.11 g
- Protein: 0.65 g

Side Effects

Excessive amount of vitamin K may affect blood clotting. So, it's advisable to consume reasonable amount of cucumber since it contains a lot vitamin K.

Some allergies associated with the consumption of cucumber include swelling and hives. Some people also report of difficult breathing. So, watch out for these signs.

NOTE

Chayote

Scientific Name: *Sechium edule*

Overview

Chayote originated from Mexico and many parts of Latin America. Now it's grown all over the world. It's also known as choko or mirliton. It is mainly used when cooked.

Almost all part of this pear-shaped plant is edible, including the root, leaves, stem, and seeds. It contains loads of nutrients that can help transform and keep the body healthy.

Major Compounds

Potassium, vitamin C, magnesium, folate, manganese, vitamin K, vitamin

B-6, zinc, quercetin, myricetin, morin, kaempferol

Health benefits

Promotes Heart Health: according to researchers, some chayote compounds help to reduce blood pressure and improve blood flow.

Also, Myricetin which is provided by the body helps to reduce the level of cholesterol in the body. Moreover, taking fiber-rich foods helps to lower the risk of heart disease - chayote is one of the fiber-rich foods.

Blood Sugar Control: the fiber content of chayote helps to promote insulin sensitivity and regulation of blood sugar.

Support Healthy Pregnancy: The folate provided by chayote helps to lower the risk of miscarriage during pregnancy.

Anticancer: the myricetin in chayote has a strong anticancer property which helps to fight against cancer.

Anti-Aging: Chayote is loaded with a high amount of antioxidants which help to protect the body cells against oxidative damage. Also, since vitamin C is verily vital in the production of collagen, the high amount of vitamin C in chayote ensures the skin stays firm and youthful.

Prevents Liver Disease: Excessive deposits of fats in the liver leads to fatty liver disease. Test tube and animal studies suggest that chayote extract can help to protect the liver by preventing the accumulation of fats in the liver.

Support Digestion: The fiber and flavonoids from chayote keep the digestive tract healthy as they keep the digestive enzymes in the gut healthy and remove wastes from the digestive tract, respectively.

How To Use

Chayote is mainly used when cooked, roasted, steamed, or fried. You can also eat it raw by adding it to your salads and smoothies.

pg. 112

You can add it to stews, soups, casserole dishes.

Nutrition fact

Per 100g

- Calories: 19
- Fat: 0.1g
- Cholesterol: 0mg
- Sodium: 2mg
- Potassium: 125mg
- Carbs: 4.5g
- Fiber: 1.7g
- Sugar: 1.7 g
- Protein: 0.8 g

Side Effects

Allergic reactions

NOTE

Bell Pepper

Scientific Name: *Capsicum annuum*

Overview

Bell peppers are 5% carbs and 94% water, with minute protein and fats.

Native to Central America, Mexico, and South America, it is cultivated in warm climate and moist soil of about 70 - 84F temperature.

It does not burn strongly like other peppers because it does not produce lipophilic chemical, capsaicin, that is responsible for the burning sensation from peppers.

Bell peppers have different colors including orange, yellow, red, and green (when unripe).

Major Compounds

Potassium, vitamins c, b-6, e, a, and k1, folate, capsanthin, violaxanthin, lutein, quercetin, luteolin,

Health benefits

Eye Health: the carotenoids, lutein and zeaxanthin, provided in large amounts by bell peppers protect the retina from oxidative damage.

Prevention Of Anemia: Iron deficiency is the major cause of weakness and tiredness of the body which is a result of the blood not being able to carry enough oxygen.

The vitamin C provided by the bell pepper promotes the absorption of iron into the body system.

How To Use

Bell pepper can be eaten raw or cooked. You can use your bell pepper in garden salads. It can be used as toppings on your cheese steaks and pizza. You can use it for your stuffed peppers. You can dry and powder it to make paprika spice.

Nutrition fact

Per 100g

- Calories: 31
- Water: 92%
- Protein: 1g
- Carbs: 6g

- Sugar: 4.2g
- Fiber: 2.1g
- Fat: 0.3g

Side Effects

Nausea, loose stools, mild burning
sensation, sneezing, stomach pain,
watery eyes

NOTE

Arugula

Scientific Name: _Eruca vesicaria_

Overview

Native to the Mediterranean, arugula is a leafy green vegetable with fresh, bitter, tart, and peppery-mustard flavor. It is popularly known is some regions as garden rocket, roquette, rucola, or colewort. It is widely used as healthy ingredient for salads.

It is super nutrition and may help the body to prevent the risk of cancer, eye damage, or osteoporosis and arthritis.

Major Compounds

Potassium, calcium, phosphorus, vitamin k, vitamin b-6, vitamin c, magnesium, sodium, thiamine, riboflavin, dietary fiber, fat, protein, vitamin a, beta-carotene, lutein zeaxanthin, niacin, vitamin e, iron,

Health Benefits

Healthy Bone: Calcium, vitamin K, magnesium, and phosphorus supplied by arugula are the major minerals for the development of strong and healthy bone. These minerals help the body to prevent any risk of osteoporosis and arthritis.

Heart Health: Arugula contains wonderful minerals to take care of the body naturally. Arugula contains high amount of potassium, vitamins and antioxidants, with moderate amount of fiber which help to protect the heart. The fiber helps the body to lower and regulate the level of cholesterol in the blood, while the potassium reduces blood pressure.

Cancer: The vitamins and antioxidants from arugula help the body to prevent the formation of cancer cells. They also protect the body cells against radical damage. This also aids anti-inflammation.

Eye Health: The high content of vitamin A, lutein and b-carotene in arugula protect and help the eyes to fight against macular degeneration.

How To Use

First rinse with cold water and dry. In addition to the leaves and seeds, it is good to know that the young seed pods, and flowers of arugula are also edible. They can be used to make salads. It can be added to soups, or used to make sauce.

Some people also use it for their pizza.

Side Effects

Some possible side effects with excessive consumption of arugula include abdominal cramping, flatulence, and discomfort.

NOTE

Turnip Greens

Scientific Name: *Brassica rapa var. rapa*

Overview

Turnip greens are root vegetables widely cultivated worldwide as food crop. It thrives better in the temperate climates. Turnip green is known as one of the best sources of vitamins and regarded as one of the healthiest vegetables in the world.

During winter and late autumn, turnip is the most common side dish in southeastern region of United States. It'sfully packed with antioxidants, potassium, calcium, and fiber.

Major Compounds

potassium, phosphorus, magnesium, pg. 126

vitamin K, folate, vitamin C, zinc, iron, sodium, Lutein, beta-Carotene,

Health Benefits

Heart Health: Turnip contains wonderful substances to take care of the body naturally. Turnip contains high amount of potassium, fiber, vitamins and antioxidants which help to protect the heart. The fiber helps the body to lower and regulate the level of cholesterol in the blood, while the potassium is a good mineral used by the body to reduce blood pressure.

Hair and Skin Care: Vitamin C in one of the major vitamins supplied by turnip to the body. Vitamin C helps the body to build and maintain collagen.

Vitamin A is vital for all body tissues including those for skin and hair. While iron helps to stop hair loss.

Healthy Bone: Calcium, vitamin K, vitamin D, magnesium, and phosphorus supplied by turnip are the major minerals for the development of strong and healthy bone. These minerals help the body to prevent any risk of osteoporosis.

Pregnancy Care: The vitamins and minerals produced by turnip are vital to keep a healthy pregnancy. Folate in the body protects pregnant women from the risk of miscarriage.

Cancer: The vitamins and antioxidants from turnip helps them to prevent the development of cancer cells. They also protect the body cells against free radical which could cause serious damage to body cells. This also aids anti- inflammation.

Eye Health: The high content of lutein and b-carotene protects and helps fight against macular degeneration.

Diabetes: Fiber is known to help in managing type 2 diabetes as it helps to regulate blood sugar.

How To Use

First rinse with cold water, and slice as desired. Turnip can be eaten raw or cooked. You can add turnip to your salad or smoothie. It can be sauteed or boiled, and added to soups, casserole, or other dishes. Side dish for rice and beans,

Side Effects

Though turnip is a wonderful source of healthy minerals, too much consumption of it may not be healthy for the body since it contains high amount of these minerals already.

Some of the possible side effects that could be associated with the consumption of turnip include runny nose, cough, watery eyes, lip swelling and redness, sore eyes, sinus, breathing problems, etc.

NOTE

Watercress

Scientific Name: *Nasturtium officinale*

Overview

Watercress is a rapid growing flowering plant that is widely used in Europe and Asia. It is native to these two continents, but has found its wide use in other regions like the Americas. It is known to be one of the oldest vegetables on earth.

It is an aquatic plant and thus, perfect for hydroponic cultivation. It is used in different delicacies and it is highly nutritious. It can be eaten raw or cooked.

Major Compounds

potassium, calcium, vitamin K,
phosphorus, folate, magnesium,
vitamin C, vitamin A, beta-Carotene,
lutein zeaxanthin, vitamin E, riboflavin,
vitamin B-6, manganese, thiamine,
pantothenic acid, iron, sodium

Health Benefits

Heart Health: Watercress contains
high amount of potassium, vitamins
and antioxidants which may help to
keep a healthy heart. High amount of
potassium helps the body to reduce
blood pressure.

Skin Care: Vitamin C helps the body
to build and maintain collagen while
vitamin A is vital for tissue
development including those for skin.

Healthy Bone: Calcium, vitamin K, vitamin C, and phosphorus from watercress are essential minerals in the formation of strong and healthy bone. These minerals keep the bones free from osteoporosis and arthritis.

Cancer: The vitamins and antioxidants from turnip helps to prevent the buildup of cancer cells. They also protect the body cells against oxidative damage to body cells.

Eye Health: The amount of lutein and b-carotene in watercress is very high and they can help to protect the eye from macular degeneration.

Other Possible Health Benefits

Some people use watercress as a
pg. 134

short-term solution for inflammation of
the lungs, baldness, and sexual
arousal.

How To Use

Mostly used to make salads,
watercress can be used in other foods
like soup, omelet, scrambled egg,
pasta sauce. It can be added to
sandwiches, wraps, smoothies, and
juice.

Side Effects

There is no enough record on the
possible side effects of watercress. It
is advisable to use moderate amount
of

watercress, and then watch out for any possible side effects.

NOTE

Purslane

Scientific Name: *Portulaca oleracea*

Overview

Purslane is a leafy green vegetable with sour and salty taste. Wide known as weed because of its ability to survive in harsh conditions, unlike other green veggies. It is more common as edible vegetable in the Middle East, Europe, and Asia. Even the Mexicans are used to it.

It can be eaten raw as salad or used in several delicacies. Its mucilaginous property makes it perfect for soups and
stews.

Major Compounds

potassium, calcium, magnesium, phosphorus, folate, vitamin B-6, vitamin E, vitamin C, vitamin A, iron, manganese, thiamine, niacin, riboflavin, zinc

Health Benefits

Anti-inflammatory: The vitamins gotten from purslane have anti-inflammatory and antioxidant properties. These properties help to protect body cells against free radicals and thus, keep the body free from inflammation. It may also be essential for cancer prevention.

Heart Health: Purslane is one of the best sources of potassium among leafy greens. Thus, may be essential for the heart, since potassium helps to reduce blood pressure.

Skin Care: Vitamin C and E the major vitamins supplied by purslane to the body. Vitamin C is known to be vital for collagen while vitamin E plays a vital role in cell regeneration. These vitamins help to keep the skin free from blemishes.

Healthy Bone: Calcium, magnesium and phosphorus provided by purslane are essential minerals for strong and healthy bones. These minerals help to prevent and treat osteoporosis and arthritis.

How To Use
Purslane's leaves, stems, and flower

buds are very much edible and they are highly nutritious. Purslane can be used in salads and soups. It is good for stir-fries. It is good to know that the fresh young leaves are the best for use.

Some people apply fresh purslane leaf on the skin to treat burns, and other skin ailments.

Side Effects

Enough data have not been recorded on the side effects associated with the use purslane.

NOTE

Amaranth Greens

Scientific Name: *Amaranthus dubious*

Overview

Amaranth Greens are herbaceous edible leafy vegetables that are native to Mexico and Central America. In the pre-Columbian time, it is one of the healthiest staple foods cultivated by the Aztecs and Incas.

Nowadays, it's mostly cultivated in the tropical climate of Asia, Latin America, and Africa where it flowers from some to fall. In the subtropical environment, it can flower throughout the year.

In India, China, and Africa amaranth is usually cultivated as leafy-vegetable. The Europeans and

Americans cultivate amaranth for their grains.

Health Benefits

- The stems and leaves contain a healthy amount of insoluble and soluble dietary fiber. This is why it is highly recommended by dieticians for a weight loss program and control of cholesterol levels in the body.

- Amaranth leaves are known to contain no zero cholesterol and a good amount of healthy fats. The greens contain approximately 23 calories/100g.

- Amaranth greens are vital for complete wellness of the body as they contain adequate amounts of antioxidants, vitamins, phytonutrients, and minerals required by the body.

- Iron is one of the essential components for the production of red blood cells. During cellular metabolism, iron serves as a co-factor for cytochrome oxidase (oxidation-reduction enzyme). A fresh Amaranth green of about 100g carries 29% DRI of iron.

- Amaranth greens contain a high amount of potassium, even more than spinach. Potassium is a very important mineral in the cells and body fluids. It helps to regulate blood pressure and heart rate.

- It also contains high amounts of magnesium, calcium, manganese, zinc, and copper, which are vital components for the body cells.

- Like other greens, amaranth helps the body in preventing weakness of the bone, which is known as iron-deficiency anemia (osteoporosis).

How To Use

For the grain:

- Add to water twice the volume of the grain or 2.4 times the weight of the grain and boil.

For the leave:

- Separate the leaf and stem.
- Wash the leaf with cold water and gently pat dry with a tissue.
- Then chop before you use it in any recipe. It can also be used without chopping.
- Do not overcook the amaranth leaf

so you don't destroy most of its nutrients, especially the vitamins and antioxidants.

- It can be used in soups, stews, curries, and mixed vegetable dishes.
- You can also use it raw to make juice or salad.

NOTE

Avocado

Scientific Name: *Persea American*

Overview

Avocado, a fruit classified as a member of Lauraceae (a flowering plant family) is claimed to originate from south- central Mexico. It's a popular plant that is cultivated throughout the world in the Mediterranean and tropical climates.

Well known as butter fruit because of its creamy texture, avocado is a nutrient-dense fruit with a high amount of healthy monounsaturated fatty acids. It contains about 20 vitamins and minerals.

Health benefits

Nutrient-Dense: Avocado is a wonderful source of vitamins B-6, K, C, and E, folate, potassium, lutein, omega-3 fatty acid, riboflavin, pathogenic acid, niacin, magnesium, and beta-carotene.

Heart Health: a healthy cholesterol level is vital for the health of our heart. Beta-sitosterol plays a vital role in maintaining the cholesterol level that is healthy for the heart. Consuming plant sterols regularly helps a lot and avocado contain about 25mg/ounce of beta-sitosterol.

Eye Health: Lutein and zeaxanthin provided by avocado serve as antioxidant protectors in the eyes to
pg. 150

reduce damage.

Osteoporosis: Vitamin K is very vital for the bone. Vitamin K helps to reduce the loss of calcium through urinary excretion and also facilitates calcium absorption. Taking half if avocado prices us with about 25% of the daily recommendation.

Cancer: although the true mechanism on how it works is yet to be known, researchers believe that the DNA and RNA are protected against undesirable mutations by folate during cell division. This folate helps to protect against cervical, stomach, colon, and pancreatic cancer.

Pregnancy: Folate also helps during

pregnancy to reduce the risk of miscarriage and possible defects if the neural tube.

Depression: homocysteine impairs the delivery of nutrients to the brain. This substance also interferes with the production of dopamine, norepinephrine, and serotonin that controls sleep, appetite, and mood. Folate helps to prevent this homocysteine from building up.

Digestion: half of avocado contains 6-7 grams of fiber. Taking this with natural fiber helps to maintain the digestive tract and lower any risk of colon cancer.

Other health benefits of avocado
pg. 152

include detoxification, antimicrobial action, protection and treatment of chronic disease and osteoporosis.

How To Use

It's important to know that we only use avocados in our meals when it ripens. How do you know when it's ripped? Gently press the skin. If it's soft and budge, then it's ripped. If not, give it some days to ripe.

You can use your avocados in your salads and sandwich, as guacamole and dip. The avocado oil is used for cooking and also for moisturizing the skin.

NOTE

CHAPTER 4

Dr Sebi
Food List

Vegetables

- ✓ Arame
- ✓ Wild Arugula
- ✓ Bell Pepper
- ✓ Zucchini
- ✓ Chayote
- ✓ Wakame
- ✓ Dulse
- ✓ Nopales
- ✓ Cucumber
- ✓ Garbanzo Beans
- ✓ Hijiki
- ✓ Sea Vegetables
- ✓ Avocado
- ✓ Dandelion Greens
- ✓ Izote flower

and leaf
- ✓ Kale
- ✓ Cherry and Plum Tomato
- ✓ Mushrooms except Shitake
- ✓ Lettuce except iceberg
- ✓ Olives
- ✓ Nori
- ✓ Onions
- ✓ Purslane Verdolaga
- ✓ Squash
- ✓ Tomatillo
- ✓ Turnip Greens

- ✓ Amaranth
- ✓ Watercress
- ✓ Okra

Fruits

- ✓ Tamarind
- ✓ Prickly Pear
- ✓ Peaches
- ✓ Bananas
- ✓ Figs
- ✓ Prunes
- ✓ Cherries
- ✓ Berries
- ✓ Rasins
- ✓ Currants
- ✓ Pears
- ✓ Dates
- ✓ Orange

- ✓ Grapes
- ✓ Limes
- ✓ Mango
- ✓ Plums
- ✓ Apples
- ✓ Soft Jelly
- ✓ Coconuts
- ✓ Melons
- ✓ Cantaloupe
- ✓ Papayas
- ✓ Soursops

Spices and Seasonings

- ✓ Sage
- ✓ Achiote
- ✓ Sweet
- ✓ Basil
- ✓ Dill

- ✓ Habanero
- ✓ Cayenne
- ✓ Bay Leaf
- ✓ Onion Powder
- ✓ Oregano
- ✓ Pure Sea Salt
- ✓ Thyme
- ✓ Savory
- ✓ Cloves
- ✓ Tarragon
- ✓ Powdered Granulated Seaweed

Grains

- ✓ Fonio
- ✓ Spelt
- ✓ Kamut

- ✓ Rye
- ✓ Tef
- ✓ Amaranth
- ✓ Quinoa
- ✓ Wild Rice

Sugars and Sweeteners

- ✓ Sugar (gotten from dried dates)
- ✓ Agave Syrup gotten from cactus (100% Pure)

Herbal Teas

- ✓ Chamomile
- ✓ Red Raspberry
- ✓ Elderberry
- ✓ Fennel
- ✓ Burdock
- ✓ Ginger
- ✓ Tila

Oils

- ✓ Avocado Oil
- ✓ Sesame Oil
- ✓ Coconut Oil
- ✓ Grapeseed Oil
- ✓ Hempseed Oil
- ✓ Olive Oil

Nuts and Seeds

- ✓ Brazil Nuts
- ✓ Raw Sesame Seeds
- ✓ Hemp seeds
- ✓ Walnuts

OTHER BOOK BY THE SAME AUTHOR

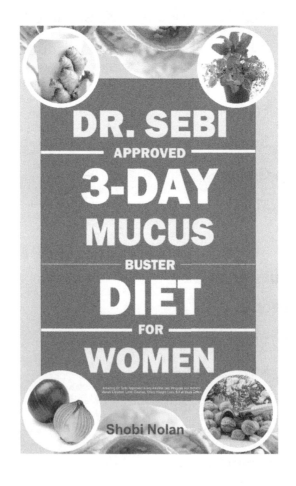

96512179R00104